CHAPTER 1: INTRODUCTION TO THE PROBLEM

Introduction

Over the past several years across the United States in healthcare, there has been an overwhelming and increasing amount of patients being medically treated at emergency departments. The main reason for this issue in healthcare is due to the bad economy, and many Americans have lost there jobs causing many families and individuals without having any finances to afford healthcare insurance or having little healthcare insurance coverage. In return, patient flow through the emergency department has been at its worst with long waits, crowding, and frustrated patients and staff members. Patient flow is a structured way in observing the patients' care process that support patients as they flow through the health care experience (Cesta, 2013). Moving patients faster through the emergency department is a crucial need, to be able to appropriately treat, address medical concerns, and provide disposition for all patients and done within a timely fashion is necessary. It is imperative for all emergency departments to identify barriers within the department that slow down the patient flow to avoid long waiting times in the waiting room which lead to negative outcomes for patients and staff members. Overcrowding and slow patient flow in the emergency department causes increase patient mortality and high risk for medical errors (Moskop, 2009). There are many different barriers within each individual emergency department that slow down patient flow, and then there are some barriers that each facility encounters as having the same problem at each facility. Regardless of the different variety of barriers, every emergency department must be able to identify these problems/issues to implement solutions and improvements for quality patient care. For the research project, the perceived thoughts of nurses based on issues/barriers in emergency departments have been collected using a questionnaire survey related to patient flow in the department.

The Problem Statement

The topic was chosen because having worked in the emergency department for several years and as an emergency department travel nurse has continuously proven at every facility how patient flow through the department is extremely slow from multiple barriers. This topic affects thousands of people in the United States of America everyday, so it is an extremely important fact that should be researched to help create solutions. In the United States there is a major shortage of access to primary care physicians, which cause higher volumes of patients receiving care in emergency departments (Cantlupe, 2012). Each healthcare facility with an emergency department functions differently and has wide ranges of certain amount of patients that visits each ED per year. All emergency departments has basic protocols and basic functions that they all share. Barriers in the emergency department that affect patient flow range from the nursing staff, laboratory department, radiology department, housekeeping department, ancillary staff, registration department, etc. Most of the departments in the hospital are linked to the emergency department that can impede the patient flow in a negative way. Patients and staff always end up being frustrated, mad, and upset about how slow patient flow through the department is. Improving patient flow through emergency departments is a necessity for patients and staff. This issue must be addressed and stop being ignored by management and leadership in hospitals. All patients deserve quality medical care within a timely fashion and in most cases this does not happen due to slow patient flow through emergency departments. Being able to assist in addressing some of these barriers may help emergency departments make improvements for the better, as it affects patients and staff greatly.

Rationale and Significance of the Study

project importance. This project is extremely important to the discipline of nursing in the emergency department. This study is being done in hopes of helping to identify nurse's awareness of issues and barriers that affect patient flow in emergency departments. Barriers and issues affect emergency departments and nursing staff every single day, which is an ongoing and continuous battle that takes place. All emergency departments must focus on areas within the organization that affects patient flow in the department. There are multiple reasons why patient flow through the ED is compromised. The research shows how significant admitted patients residing in the emergency department affects patient flow. This research is being done in hopes that emergency departments can make improvements and resolve issues to quickly move admitted patients out of the emergency department to help improve patient flow. The study shows how nurses perceive barriers/issues related to patient flow in the emergency department. To get a clear understanding of nurses thoughts and feelings on the issue at hand pertaining to the emergency department. In turn, this can help nurses become creative with ideas for improvement. Or this will show how unaware nurses are to a huge problem in emergency departments and are in need of education and understanding on the issue.

problem outline. Improving patient flow through emergency departments is crucial to prevent overcrowding and long-wait times in the waiting room. When patient flow is good and organized there is improved patient safety, improved quality of care, and improved operational efficiency (Cesta, 2013). Every staff member is involved in patient flow and each job can slow down flow through the department if not done in a timely fashion. The emergency department is a fast paced, rushed, highly tensed, and stressful department to work in which causes high burn out rates and high staff turnover rates. Identifying barriers that affect emergency department patient flow is essential to make improvements and changes to the necessary areas. Negative consequences for patients, staff, and hospital facility have proven to happen when there is slow patient flow through the emergency department. Overcrowding in emergency department waiting rooms has been proven to cause patient harm and decrease patient satisfactory scores so the need to create strategies to improve flow is great (Wiler, 2011).

background information. Due to the economy crisis over the past couple of years, the unemployment rates have been extremely high leaving many people without healthcare insurance. In turn, many Americans do not have primary care physicians so in turn they come to the emergency department for their medical needs and care. Due to this switch in healthcare, waiting rooms have been overcrowded and routinely result in long waiting periods to be seen in the emergency department. Unfortunately, ED's are overcome by problems associated with the demand for services and limitations of resources such as overcrowding, long wait times, and operational inefficiencies (Stone-Griffith, 2012). It has become essential for all emergency departments to identify barriers and resolve issues to improve patient flow.

possible causes of problem. There are many reasons within each individual emergency department that causes barriers which slow patient flow down through the department. Admitted patients in the emergency department causes decrease patient flow. The main reason for overcrowding and decrease patient flow in the emergency department is due to admitted patients (Richardson, 2009). Admitted patients in the emergency department usually takes hours waiting on an inpatient bed which in turn occupies space and beds in the ED which slows the patient flow down tremendously. This in results causes overcrowding in the waiting room and long waiting times to be seen and treated by the doctors and nursing staff. A study was done across many hospital emergency departments and it was found that the amount of admissions per day had the most correlation between the average lengths of stay in the emergency department (Lucas, 2009). There are multiple reasons why admitted patients have long waiting periods in the emergency department which are due to: no rooms available, no staffing available, dirty rooms not cleaned yet by housekeeping, and floor nursing staff stalling techniques. These are the main factors that prevent admitted patients from going to the inpatient unit in a timely fashion. An additional barrier includes waiting on the laboratory department for blood and urine results. Many times it takes up to 2 hours or more waiting for results, which is a huge factor for deciding on admissions, treatments, and diagnoses for each patient. Decreasing lab turnaround time positively and substantially affects the ED patient flow with length of stay and ED throughput (Storrow, 2008). Another area that is a barrier is the radiology department. Radiology results such as x-rays, cat scans, and ultrasound reports can take 1-2 hours or more, and it depends on if the radiologist is located at that facility or the results have to be sent electronically to a radiologist at another facility to interpret the results. These factors can slow down the patient flow in the emergency department especially if they are combined together causing wait times to increase. This is why it is so important to be able to identify barriers that slow down patient flow to make improvements to these areas.

Research Question

The research will address the following research question:

1. How do nurses perceive patient flow issues through emergency departments?

Definition of Terms

ED – abbreviation for emergency department. An emergency department is a medical treatment facility which is mainly located in a hospital or primary care center that specializes in caring for patients with acute illnesses without an appointment arriving by either an ambulance or by other individual means (Wikipedia, 2014).

Summary

Patient flow in emergency departments is definitely an issue and is in need of improvements. The only way improvements can be made and initiated will be done by first identifying the causes of impediment of patient flow. After these multiple barriers have been identified then staff members and leadership members can come together and collaborate what the best solution to each individual barrier will be. Then when a solution has been recognized the next step will be to initiate a run trial to observe and see if it will fix or improve the problem.

Improving patient flow is a wide spread problem throughout the United States. This problem can be improved greatly with a little effort and research. Patients deserve quality medical care in the United States and becoming a team of healthcare professionals we are capable of providing this type of care and service.

CHAPTER 2:
LITERATURE REVIEW

Introduction

Improving patient flow through the emergency is definitely a problem due to multiple barriers within the department and outside the department. Systemic inefficiencies and incentives in hospitals cause ED overcrowding and negative outcomes for patients (Handel, 2010). Many problematic factors lie outside of the emergency department, which is out of ED staff control, but there are still inside department changes that can take effect for improvements. The literature review will provide information that supports patient flow being a problem in the emergency department. The literature review will also provide insight on multiple factors causing the issues and ways for improvement. There have been many reports and research done on improving patient flow, some methods have succeeded and some have not been as successful as others. The important thing is to continue striving for methods that help all emergency departments in the United States.

keywords. Keywords that were used to search for the literature review included: admitted patients, admission patients, wait-times, overcrowding, delays, slow, decompression, and dispositions.

Emergency Department Overcrowding

The institute of Medicine has declared that emergency departments in the United States have become a "national epidemic" (Horwitz, 2010). Overcrowding in the emergency department is the main reason for the need to improve patient flow through the department. About 96% of ED directors across the United States report that overcrowding is a problem and 28% report that this occurs on a daily basis (Felton, 2011). Overcrowding occurs when the demand for emergency department services exceeds the available supply or the lack to move patients to inpatient areas (Barrett, 2012). Overcrowding causes many issues and problems with patients, staff, and facility. Poor patient care, frustrated patients, increased costs, potential harm, and stress on patients and staff is caused by overcrowding (Cantlupe, 2013). This is a problem not only in the waiting room of the emergency department but also an issue in the actual department when patients are placed in hallways and chairs instead of being in a room for treatment for privacy. There are multifactor causes of crowding in emergency departments (Schiff, 2011). One reason for crowding in the emergency department is the lack of being able to move patients out of the ED in an efficient and timely manner, which requires the cooperation between the inpatient units in the health care facility (McClelland, 2011). Admitted patients occupying space in the emergency department until an inpatient bed become available is the reason for ED overcrowding (Viccellio, 2009).

      negative consequences. Many negative consequences arise in the emergency department when it comes to having overcrowding. Reports of emergency department crowding are high with negative effects such as ambulance diversion, prolonged patient wait times, high patient complaints, decreased physician productivity, decreased staff satisfaction, and suboptimal clinical outcomes (Stone-Griffith, 2012). Negative consequences involve not only patients but also staff members and the facility that the emergency department resides in. Negative effects include quality of care such as wrong medications, wrong or over-utilization of medications and treatments, misuse of products and personnel resources, and delays in care process like core measures (Cesta, 2013). There are adverse effects of ED overcrowding for clinical outcomes, which include mortality, time to treatment with patients that have time-sensitivity conditions, and many others (Bernstein, 2009). Long wait times in emergency departments cause bad patient and employee satisfaction and also aide to patients leaving without being seen by a physician (Jarousse, 2011). These negative issues also include finical strains on the facility and patients. When patients have bad clinical outcomes they end up having to receive longer extended treatments in hospitals and some have to receive higher acuity care and all this cost the facility and/or patient more money. Healthcare leaders recognize that due to overcrowding in emergency departments safety has become a major concern with patients (Cantlupe, 2012). This issue also causes problems with poor staff retention and high turnover rates in the emergency department. Nursing staff ends up being burnt out quickly, working in this department, which causes increased finical burden on the facility by having to train new staff constantly to replace old staff that has left or transferred out of the department.

Emergency Department Admissions

To improve patient flow through emergency departments admitted patients residing in the department should be expedited to inpatient units. These patients continue to be an ongoing problem during high peak times in the emergency department. They occupy space and beds that are needed for ill patients waiting in the waiting area that have yet to be seen by a physician. Increased inpatient length of stay and high inpatient cost is related to delays of admitted patients in the emergency department (Huang, 2010). Diminished quality of patient care and poor patient outcomes are related to excessive amount of admitted patients in the emergency department (Richardson, 2009). A facility not being able to admit emergency department patients in a timely fashion to inpatient unit is referred to as access block. Access block is a serious issue that contributes to 20%-30% excess mortality rates each year and attributes to compromising patient safety and quality of care (Fatovich, 2009). In a single variable study done showed that there is a strong correlation between emergency department admissions and emergency department length of stay (Lucas, 2009). An observation discovered that number of emergency department admissions and hospital occupancy rate was positively associated with ED length of stay (McCarthy, 2009). There are multiple avenues and techniques that can be done to implement with aiding in moving admitted patients quickly to inpatient units and out of the emergency department. A study was done for communication improvement to reduce the length of stay in the ED for admitted patients which included fax reports to inpatient units and a bed coordinator position to monitor occupancy rates with the floors and communicate with the emergency department and address needs for admissions. This improved communication with speed of admissions and effectively decreasing ED crowding and improved ED patient flow (McHugh, 2013). Another strategy implemented in a study was used to predict or anticipate inpatient unit bed demand for ED admissions. The model is called logit-linear regression model and it allowed bed managers to plan for peak and high demand early enough to help better prioritize clinical activities, discharge patients in timely manner, and prepare room assignments for patients as needed (Peck, 2012). There are several different techniques that can be used to help with decompressing admitted patients in the emergency department to inpatient units to improve patient flow through the department. Unfortunately, there are times when there are no available beds in the hospital and the occupancy level is high which is when ED admit patients end up residing in the ED for a night or more until inpatients are discharge to open up an available room. This is an issue out of the ED's control, but hospital administration and leadership should analysis and observe these times to come up with a possible solution to this problem.

Best Practices Research

There are multiple avenues that facilities have attempted to take for patient flow improvements. Each facility has different available resources and should alter each technique strategy for their facility and based on their individual needs. Facilities should continue to find ways for improvements to patient flow if one or more methods become a failure. Opportunities to improve patient flow in the emergency department are many, and hospital facilities that engage staff in improvement efforts can derive substantial cost, quality, and increase patient satisfaction benefits (Johnson, 2012). A study was done in 6 emergency departments that included either a Nurse Practitioner or a Physician Assistant involved in direct patient care or indirectly patient care. In this study it was concluded that it greatly improved patient flow and significantly reduced length of stays and reduced patients who left without being seen (Ducharme, 2009). The majority of emergency departments use a Nurse Practitioner or Physician Assistant or both in fast track areas in the department. These patients usually have acuity levels of 4 and 5, which are non-urgent patients that can be quickly seen and discharged in a short time. Utilizing a fast track for patients in the emergency department results in fewer patients leaving without being seen, shorter waiting time, and shorter length of stay (Oredsson, 2011). Using fast tacks in emergency departments is related to a definite increase in throughput and lowers the time it takes waiting for a bed in the department (Peck, 2010). An additional excellent practice that can contribute to improvements is implementing an admission pending unit, clinical decision unit, or observation unit. These types of units can create an area for admitted patients outside the ED when inpatient units are full and provide continuing evaluation and treatment (Moskop, 2009). This will help decompress the emergency department tremendously along with continuing to provide appropriate quality care for admitted patients. Many times when admit patients wait in the ED, the ED nurse is mainly focusing on other acutely ill patients being assigned and quickly completing orders such as stat blood draws, medications, and other stat test that may need to be done on patients. So with the ED nurse caring for new patients being assigned, admit patient orders are not being initiated unless it is a stat order as it would have been initiated if they were on an inpatient unit. So this delays treatment for the admit patients. These are just a few of the best practices for the majority emergency departments, but there are among many more that can be implemented for improving patient flow.

Summary

In conclusion this literature review presents abundant amount of evidence dealing with the issues related to patient flow through the emergency department. Problems arising from patient flow in the emergency department are caused by many barriers, which lie within the department and also a systematic facility issues that contributes. For nurses to become involved and active in improvements first they must be aware of these issues happening in the emergency department. The research study that has been conducted on nurses will help in providing understanding and perceived thoughts of barriers/issues related to patient flow in emergency departments. There are multiple avenues to take for implementing improvement strategies to help improve patient flow with the assistance of identifying the main causes of barriers. The fact is that improving patient flow will help prevent overcrowding in the emergency department, which leads to negative outcomes for patient, staff, and facility.

CHAPTER 3: METHODOLOGY

Introduction

     This chapter will give insight of the methodology details of the research project. A quantitative study was chosen involving the understanding of nurses perceived thoughts involving issues and barriers' pertaining to patient flow in emergency departments. This methodology will provide details of the processes it took to plan and implement this research study.

Setting

     The study was done on an online website using a survey questionnaire. The online website used to send out the questionnaires was SurveyMonkey which is a well known and a trusted company for Institutional Review Board (IRB) approved graduate data analysis studies. The researcher used SurveyMonkeys' database to send out the questionnaire by emailing nurse participants the link to access the survey questions. The nurse recipients clicked on the secure link and begin completing the survey questionnaire.

Participants

     The participants for the study included 20 random nurses from SurveyMonkey database. These nurses had all different types of work background and experiences but all worked and lived in the United States. Work background experiences included emergency department, medical surgical unit, intensive care unit, behavioral health unit, telemetry unit, coronary care unit, transitional intensive care unit, primary care offices/

specialist offices, home health care, health department clinics, nursing home facilities, and hospice facilities. The nurses had all different years of experience and all different levels of education. The different levels of education included diploma degrees, associate degrees, bachelor degrees, master degrees, and doctrine degrees. The variety titles that these nurses hold included License Practical Nurses/License Vocational Nurses, Registered Nurses, Nurse Practitioners, and Doctor of Nursing Practice/PhD in Nursing. The variety levels of experience included novice, advance beginner, competent, proficient, and experts working in nursing. Study participants with all ethnicities and all economical situations that included lower class, middle class, and upper class. All races were apart of the study that did include Whites, Blacks, Hispanics, Asians, and American Indian. They have all different cultures and learning styles. Ages of 18 years and older and males and females was part of the study.

Research Design

For the research project, the non-experimental quantitative method was used. Quantitative research method is a controlled, systematic, empirical, and serious investigation of hypothetical propositions among presumed relations with natural phenomena using numbers (Tappen, 2010). A simple descriptive design will be implemented which will focus on a certain population or a single group (Tappen, 2010). The single focus group was nurses from a probability random sample. In using this type of research method and design, a survey questionnaire has been created in answering the research question. The survey questionnaire included 8 questions to gain knowledge of nurses perceived thoughts on issues related to patient flow through emergency departments. The survey questionnaire is located on the Internet using SurveyMonkey. This research method was adopted because it can accurately show details of barriers in the emergency department and nurses thoughts concerning these issues within the department. Being able to collect all responses from multiple nurses and using numbers to identify the majority opinions assisted in answering the research questions. The most basic survey designs are mainly used to obtain answers, which can be tallied and reported numerically (Tappen, 2010).

Description of Instruments or Tools

The evaluation method being used in the study is a non-experimental quantitative method. The researcher chose a quantitative research method study to provide visual statistical data, with the manipulation of numbers to depict an expression of nurses perceived thoughts about issues and barriers related to patient flow in emergency departments. Quantitative research methods are used to provide the collection and analysis of numerical data to describe the phenomena of interest in a way that will have little personal interaction with the participants (Mills, 2011). The instrument that was used to collect the data was a laptop computer using an Internet source. The main tool/instrument being utilized in the study is an 8-question survey to express issues and barriers pertaining to patient flow in emergency departments and receive input from nurses about their thoughts and opinions on this topic of chose (see Appendix C). The Internet source was used to access SurveyMonkey, to create and distribute the survey questionnaire to participants. The survey questionnaire was distributed by SurveyMonkey database to 20 random nurses. The questions had either a multiple answer responses or a simple yes and no response for each question. After the responses were collected from participants the use of a pie and bar chart was implemented to show the results in an aggregated form. The pie and bar chart showed each answer in percentage form.

reliability and validity. Reliability and validity are very important aspects used to evaluate quality quantitative studies (Tappen, 2010). Reliability focuses on research measures, which can be signified in a variety of ways that can include consistency, repeatability, stability, predictability, homogeneity, agreement, and reproducibility (Tappen, 2010). The research project is consistent, by using the same method to distribute the survey questionnaire to participants by email, at the same time and day, and using the same analysis ensured consistency. SurveyMonkey is responsible and competent in distributing to participants and provide analysis of data. SurveyMonkey is a well-known and reliable company specifically focused in assisting individuals with designing, collecting, and analysis data using surveys, which has been done many of times repeatedly for variety types of organizations, events, campaigns, research projects, etc. Validity is basically the extent at which the researcher tool used is used for its intended purpose (Tappen, 2010). The researcher created the survey questionnaire after the literature review of at least 25-30 references related to the research topic. All survey questions stayed focused and directly based on the literature review in dealing with patient flow issues/barriers related to emergency departments.

Data Collection

The data collection process was implemented through the use of SurveyMonkey. Using a non-experimental quantitative research method, the researcher created an 8-question survey questionnaire in SurveyMonkey, which also included an informed consent provided on the first page, and then the survey was distributed to participants. SurveyMonkey database was used to distribute the survey questionnaire to 20 random nurse participants. SurveyMonkey emailed participants with an attached link to the survey questionnaire. If participants choose the option to disagree to informed consent, they will be instructed not to continue in taking the survey questionnaire. After participants took the survey questionnaire, the responses were readily available to be viewed by the researcher. Responses by the participants were automatically presented in a pie and bar chart representing the percentage of each individual answer for each question from the total of participants. The researcher had access to each individual participant response for each question. The participants received the survey questionnaire at the same time and day and had an open period of 7 days to take the survey. After the 7-day period all results were analyzed and presented in a pie and bar chart form. The integrity of the data collection was maintained in an intact state. No questions from individual response was deleted or impaired to achieve a certain outcome for questions. Data that was collected was maintained in SurveyMonkey with a username and password sign-in access. Data collected visible on research computerized written report was accessed only by a laptop computer with a username and password sign-in access.

Data Analysis

The data analysis for the quantitative research method project used basic division and multiplication. In an aggregated form, all answers from participants were presented as a percentage to reveal results. To calculate the percentage for each response answer, the following was used: the number of participants that chose that answer divided by the number of all participants multiplied times 100 calculated the percentage results. This was done for each yes and no answer and multiple-choice answer. Then, the results were presented in a pie and bar chart form. The pie and bar chart was shown for each question, with each answer percentage, representing the combination of all participants. In doing so, this showed the majority responses to the questions based on nurses' thoughts. Using percentages, as a statistical data represented an expressive form of numbers showing how nurses perceive issues/barriers related to patient flow issues in emergency departments.

Human Subjects Protection

Human subject protection is very important to be maintained for the study. The very first step taken was to obtain a certification from The National Institutes of Health (NIH) for the completion of a Web-based training course "Protecting Human Research Participants" (see Appendix A). The researcher decided to perform the research study at SurveyMonkey. Then the research had to gain permission from two different Institutional Review Boards before proceeding with the study. The first organization was an online web-based company at SurveyMonkey. To obtain permission from SurveyMonkey, there were requirements for the informed consent, confidentiality guidelines, all survey questions allow "no response", and participants given the option to withdraw from the survey at any time. With agreement of these terms and conditions, then the researcher was able to obtain an official approval letter from the Institutional Review Board (IRB) at SurveyMonkey to conduct the research study (see Appendix B). The second organization for approval was Western Governors University. The Institutional Review Board from Western Governors University granted approval for the researcher to conduct the study. Both organizations required an agreement for an informed consent to be included for approval. The informed consent had to contain no penalty for withdraw from study at any time and indicate participants confidentiality maintained. The data was stored on a username and password access laptop computer only in possession of the researcher and online access to data with a username and password account. SurveyMonkey has a very safe and secure website that is recognized for using VeriSign, TRUSTe, McAfee, and the Better Business Bureau. Data results and any confidential information were not printed.

Summary

Every step in this quantitative research project has been analyzed and researched to begin with the data collection process. Approvals and consents have been granted and implemented and all precautionary steps have been outlined. This online data collection research study approach will open up opportunities to gather opinions of all types of nurses across the United States that could not have been achieved if the researcher had focused on one healthcare facility. In using this type of research model for the quantitative study of chose, will heed more of a realistic look at nurses' opinions concerning this topic.

CHAPTER 4: FINDINGS

Overview

The general purpose of the this study was to understand nurses perceived thoughts pertaining to issues/barriers related to patient flow through emergency departments. A quantitative research study was implemented using an 8-question survey questionnaire distributed to nurse participants to answer. This chapter will outline the analysis of data and results with an interpretation of what the study outcome really means.

Analysis of Data

The survey questionnaire was electronically distributed through SurveyMonkeys' database system. It was distributed to a random number of nurses with a total of 20 nurse participants that fully participated and completed the entire questionnaire. Barriers and issues pertaining to patient flow through the emergency department were used in creating the survey questions.

Figure 1 represents the first survey question in a pie chart. This question is straightforward asking nurses do they feel patient flow through emergency departments is a problem. 100% of participants agreed that patient flow is a problem in emergency departments.

Figure 1. Survey Question Number One Results

Figure 2 represents the second survey question in a pie chart. Asking participants how likely is it that the cause of emergency department overcrowding is from decreased patient flow through the department. 55% responded very likely, 25% responded moderately likely, 10% responded slightly likely, and 10% responded not at all likely that overcrowding is from decreased patient flow. 90% of participants voted that it is likely that overcrowding is caused by decreased patient flow through the emergency department.

Figure 2. Survey Question Number Two Results

Figure 3 represents the third survey question in a pie chart. This ask participants do they think the lack of medical insurance from patients related to the bad economy and high unemployment rates is the reason for patient flow problems in emergency departments. 90% of participants agreed that the statement is true. 60% responded very true, 15% responded moderately true, 15% responded slightly true, and 10% responded not at all true.

Figure 3. Survey Question Number Three Results

Figure 4 represents the fourth survey question in a pie chart. This question asks do the nurses think that the patient flow problem lies only within the emergency department. 85% of the participants answered no. Only 15% answered yes that the problems only lies within the emergency department.

Figure 4. Survey Question Number Four Results

Figure 5 represents survey question five in a pie chart. This question asks basically does admitted patients in the emergency department slow down patient flow. 95% of participants agreed that admitted patients does affect patient flow through the department. 70% responded extremely influential, 20% responded moderately influential, 5% slightly influential, and 5% responded not at all influential.

Figure 5. Survey Question Number Five Results

Figure 6 represents survey question six in a pie chart. This is asking nurses, can hospital census affect patient flow through the department. 95% of participants stated yes, hospital census does affect patient flow in the ED. 5% of participants responded no.

Figure 6. Survey Question Number Six Results

Figure 7 represents survey question seven in a pie chart. This asks nurses, can decreased patient flow negatively affect quality care and patient safety. 100% of participants stated that yes quality care and patient safety can be affected. 50% responded always, 20% responded often, 25% responded sometimes, and 5% responded rarely.

Figure 7. Survey Question Number Seven Results

Figure 8 represents survey question eight in a bar chart. This is asking nurses which barrier(s) is the most likely cause of decreased patient flow and for them to select all that apply. 90% responded admitted patients in ED, 45% responded waiting on lab results, 45% responded waiting on radiology results, 70% responded not enough inpatient beds, 50% responded not enough staff available, 10% responded with giving there own specific response to barriers.

Table 1 represents the comments made by participants from question 8. 10% of participants had a specific written barrier comment that was included. One participant responded "patient's that do not need to be seen in emergency setting" is a barrier. The second participant responded "waiting on MD" is a barrier.

Figure 8. Survey Question Number Eight Results

Table 1. Question 8 Part 2 Specific Responses

Part 2: Which barrier(s) is the most likely cause of negative effects on patient flow through emergency departments? (Other, please specify)	
Number of Responses	**Comments**
1	Patients that do not need to be seen in emergency setting.
1	Waiting on MD.

Results and Interpretation

The survey questions were created using the literature review based on patient flow issues/barriers in emergency departments. In turn, this quantitative research study provided visual statistical data, with the manipulation of numbers to depict an expression of nurses perceived thoughts about issues and barriers related to patient flow in emergency departments. Based on the outcome from the nurses completing the survey questionnaire, all participants understand that patient flow is an issue through emergency departments. One huge barrier that disrupts the flow through the department is admitted patients residing in the emergency department. There were a few questions that focused on admitted patients affecting patient flow, and at least 90% of the nurse participants agreed that admitted patients affect the flow through emergency departments. The majority of participants agreed that decrease patient flow could have negative affects such as overcrowding, poor quality care, and negative affects on patient safety. Most nurse participants were able to identify barriers affecting patient flow and understood that the problem does not only reside within the department but a systematic problem within the entire facility. 90% of participants agreed that results from the bad economy and high employment rates have affected patient flow in emergency departments. There were only 10% or fewer participants that did not completely understand or agree with some of the barriers and causes from patient flow issues in emergency departments.

With the use of the survey questionnaire, the research question was answered. The research question was as follows: How do nurses perceive patient flow issues through emergency departments? The nurses perceive that patient flow is definitely an issue in emergency departments and there are multiple barriers and issues that impede the flow through the department. They comprehend the major issue with admitted patients affecting flow through the department. They also understand how this can negatively affect patients. Nurses are aware that the problem does not only reside within the ED but a systematic issue.

Summary

In conclusion, this quantitative research project turned out good with very informative results from the 20 nurse participants. The researcher was able to provide statistical data, represented in an expressive form of numbers showing how nurses perceive issues and barriers related to patient flow in emergency departments. All of the participants agreed that patient flow is an issue and the majority understood what barriers affected patient flow, which assisted the researcher in answering the research question.

Chapter 5: Discussion and Conclusion

Introduction

The general purpose of this research was to discuss patient flow issues and barriers pertaining to the emergency department. An investigation was done in how nurses perceive issues and barriers related to patient flow in emergency departments. In this chapter, the researcher will provide insight in a discussion, implications, limitations, and recommendations related to the research study.

Discussion

The general purpose of the research study was to bring about insight dealing with patient flow through emergency departments. The research studied the perceived thoughts of nurses based on issues and barriers related to patient flow in emergency departments. The literature review provided an abundance amount of information regarding barriers and issues related to emergency departments and ways for best practices to improve patient flow. In using SurveyMonkeys' database an 8-question survey questionnaire was distributed to 20 nurses via email to obtain results. In the findings, the following research question was answered: How do nurses perceive patient flow issues through emergency departments? The findings suggested that 100% of the nurses perceived that patient flow through emergency departments is definitely an issue. The majority of nurses were aware of the different types of barriers and issues that impeded the flow through emergency departments. They understood negative effects on patients this can have and that this is systematic issue within the facility.

Implications

The main implication of the research study implied that patient flow is a problem in emergency departments across the United States. Based on the research, admitted patients residing in emergency departments, waiting on inpatient beds causes a major barrier with patient flow through the department. The data analysis results have proven that nurses are aware of this ongoing problem with patient flow in emergency departments. With this knowledge, nurses should be able to collaborate with different ideas for development and growth pertaining to patient flow issues. The strength in this study was providing an easy and convenient response from participants. This was an easy quick survey questionnaire with participants being able to complete the survey from any device with an Internet connection that could have included smart phone, laptop, tablet, iPad, etc. It was easy to distribute to participants and received a quick response from participants.

Limitations

There was some weakness with the study. The amount of responses from nurses were only 20, more participants would have been ideal to get a better perception of more random nurses opinions. The next weakness in the study was involving nurses that may have never actually worked in the emergency department may have skewed the results. To be able to identify with an issue it would have been more appropriate to align participants that have worked in an emergency department in some point of there nursing career to give an opinion pertaining to the issue. There most likely would not have been a small percentage of the participants that did not agree with some of the barriers and issues pertaining to patient flow in emergency departments, if all participants had actually worked in an emergency department.

Recommendations

There are a few possible solutions based on the results of the project. A major solution is to move admitted patients out of the emergency department as soon as possible to prevent occupying space and beds from patients that are in the waiting room, which in turns improves patient flow. Other inpatient departments will have to be apart of the plan to have open rooms available when there is a need from the emergency department to move a patient quickly to decompress the department. An uncontrollable solution from healthcare providers is for everybody to get medical insurance. The lack of medical insurance causes people with minor problems and long term untreated conditions to come to the emergency department, which could have been prevented if they had a primary medical physician. As of 2014 due to obamacare this can be implemented to hopefully have a major improvement with patient flow in emergency departments. Other solutions include faster lab and radiology results, so the physician can implement a plan to treat and discharge or admit the patient. This will provide a quick turnover rate with patients to prevent overcrowding in the emergency department waiting room.

Areas of the topic that could be furthered investigated could be improving patient flow through emergency departments. More of an in-depth investigation of improvement strategies and plans pertaining to the problem would be informative. Even though the researcher did some research on improvement strategies a deeper study could have been done on that particular part. This would bring about enlightenment of multiple options for different facilities to choose from that would fit their own individual needs. A questionnaire could be sent to at least 50 currently or recently working ER nurse participants that would include questions related to improvement patient flow strategies related to the emergency department. This could be a really good future research study based off the researchers' findings and limitations that followed.

If the research study were done again in the future there would be a couple of things that the researcher would alter. First, the survey questionnaire would only be distributed to nurses that are currently or recently (within a year) working in an emergency department. Second, at least 50 participants or more would have been obtained to get a stronger viewpoint from ER nurses. This would have achieved a stronger and solid data analysis finding.

Conclusions

In conclusion, research studies will always have pros and cons. Even though there were better routes and implications that the researcher could have taken during the research project the results came out good, considering. In the findings the research question was answered appropriately. Based on the entire research there was a great deal of knowledge and information gathered to understand the problem with patient flow in emergency departments across the United States. The results provided several possible solutions to the research problem. This will hopefully bring about logical discussions for more extensive improvements for the problem at hand from the participants and readers of this research project.

References

Barrett, L., Ford, S., & Ward-Smith, P. (2012). A bed management strategy for
    overcrowding in the emergency department. Nursing Economic$, 30(2), 82-86.

Bernstein, S., Aronsky, D., Duseja, R., Epstein, S., Handel, D., Hwang, U., & ... Asplin, B.
    (2009). The effect of emergency department crowding on clinically oriented outcomes. Academic Emergency Medicine: Official Journal Of The Society For Academic Emergency Medicine, 16(1), 1-10. doi:10.1111/j.1553-2712.2008.00295.x

Cantlupe, J. (2013). Keys to better flow, better \are in EDs. Healthleaders Magazine,
    16(4), 44-51.

Cantlupe, J. (2012). The focus on flow. Healthleaders Magazine, 15(5), 22-26.

Cesta, T. (2013). Managing length of stay using patient flow - Part 1. hospital case
    management, 21(2), 19-22.

Ducharme, J., Alder, R. J., Pelletier, C., Murray, D., & Tepper, J. (2009). The impact on
    patient flow after the integration of nurse practitioners and physician assistants in 6 Ontario emergency departments. CJEM, 11(5), 455-61.

Felton, B., Reisdorff, E., Krone, C., & Laskaris, G. (2011). Emergency department
    overcrowding and inpatient boarding: A statewide glimpse in time. Academic Emergency Medicine: Official Journal Of The Society For Academic Emergency Medicine, 18(12), 1386-1391. doi:10.1111/j.1553-2712.2011.01209.x

Handel, D. A., Hilton, J. A., Ward, M. J., Rabin, E., Zwemer Jr, F. L., & Pines, J.
    M. (2010). Emergency department throughput, crowding, and financial outcomes for hospitals. Academic Emergency Medicine, 17(8), 840-847.

Horwitz, L. I., Green, J., & Bradley, E. H. (2010). US emergency department performance on
>   wait time and length of visit. Annals of emergency medicine, 55(2), 133-141.

Huang, Q., Thind, A., Dreyer, J., & Zaric, G. (2010). The impact of delays to admission from
>   the emergency department on inpatient outcomes. BMC
>   Emergency Medicine, 1016. doi:10.1186/1471-227X-10-16

Jarousse, L. (2011). ED throughput: A key to patient safety. H&HN: Hospitals &
>   Health Networks, 85(8), 33-39.

Johnson, M. (2012). Improving patient flow through the emergency department. Journal
>   Of Healthcare Management, 57(4), 236-243.

Lucas, R., Farley, H., Twanmoh, J., Urumov, A., Olsen, N., Evans, B., & Kabiri, H.
>   (2009). Emergency department patient flow: The influence of hospital census variables on emergency department length of stay. Academic Emergency Medicine: Official Journal Of The Society For Academic Emergency Medicine, 16(7), 597-602. doi:10.1111/j.1553-2712.2009.00397.x

McCarthy, M. L., Zeger, S. L., Ding, R., Levin, S. R., Desmond, J. S., Lee, J., & Aronsky, D.
>   (2009). Crowding delays treatment and lengthens emergency department length of stay, even among high-acuity patients. Annals of emergency medicine, 54(4), 492-503.

McClelland, M., Lazar, D., Sears, V., Wilson, M., Siegel, B., & Pines, J. (2011). The past,
>   present, and future of urgent matters: Lessons learned from a decade of emergency department flow improvement. Academic Emergency Medicine: Official Journal Of The Society For Academic Emergency Medicine, 18(12), 1392-1399. doi:10.1111/j.1553-2712.2011.01229.x

McHugh, M., Van Dyke, K., Howell, E., Adams, F., Moss, D., & Yonek, J. (2013). Changes in
>   patient flow among five hospitals participating in a learning

collaborative. *Journal For Healthcare Quality: Official Publication Of The National Association For Healthcare Quality*, *35*(1), 21-29. doi:10.1111/j.1945-1474.2011.00163.x

Mills, G. E. (2011). Action research: A guide for the teacher researcher, 4/e, VitalSource

for Western Governors University [VitalSouce bookshelf version]. Retrieved from http://online.vitalsource.com/books/9781256819336/id/ch01bx3

Moskop, J. C., Sklar, D. P., Geiderman, J. M., Schears, R. M., & Bookman, K. J. (2009).

Emergency department crowding, part 1—concept, causes, and moral consequences. Annals of emergency medicine, 53(5), 605-611.

Moskop, J. C., Sklar, D. P., Geiderman, J. M., Schears, R. M., & Bookman, K. J. (2009).

Emergency department crowding, part 2—barriers to reform and strategies to overcome them. Annals of emergency medicine, 53(5), 612-617.

Oredsson, S., Jonsson, H., Rognes, J., Lind, L., Goransson, K. E., Ehrenberg, A., ... &

Farrohknia, N. (2011). A systematic review of triage-related interventions to improve patient flow in emergency departments. *Scand J Trauma Resusc Emerg Med*, *19*(1), 43.

Peck, J., Benneyan, J., Nightingale, D., & Gaehde, S. (2012). Predicting emergency

department inpatient admissions to improve same-day patient flow. *Academic Emergency Medicine: Official Journal Of The Society For Academic Emergency Medicine*, *19*(9), E1045-E1054. doi:10.1111/j.1553-2712.2012.01435.x

Peck, J. S., & Kim, S. G. (2010). Improving patient flow through axiomatic design

of hospital emergency departments. CIRP Journal of Manufacturing Science and Technology, 2(4), 255-260.

Richardson, D. B., & Mountain, D. (2009). Myths versus facts in emergency department

overcrowding and hospital access block. Medical Journal of

Australia, 190(7), 369.

Schiff, G. (2011). System dynamics and dysfunctionalities: Levers for overcoming
emergency department overcrowding. Academic Emergency Medicine: Official Journal Of The Society For Academic Emergency Medicine, 18(12), 1255-1261. doi:10.1111/j.1553-2712.2011.01225.x

Stone-Griffith, S., Englebright, J., Cheung, D., Korwek, K., & Perlin, J. (2012). Data-driven
process and operational improvement in the emergency department: The ED dashboard and reporting application. Journal Of Healthcare Management / American College Of Healthcare Executives, 57(3), 167-180.

Storrow, A., Zhou, C., Gaddis, G., Han, J., Miller, K., Klubert, D., & ... Aronsky, D.
(2008). Decreasing lab turnaround time improves emergency department
throughput and decreases emergency medical services diversion: A simulation
model. Academic Emergency Medicine: Official Journal Of The Society For
Academic Emergency Medicine, 15(11), 1130-1135. doi:10.1111/j.1553-
2712.2008.00181.x

Tappen, R. (2010). Advanced nursing research: From theory to practice (1st ed). Jones &
Bartlett Learning. Retrieved from http://online.vitalsource.com/books/9781449679613/id/ch06lev2sec5

Viccellio, A., Santora, C., Singer, A. J., Thode Jr, H. C., & Henry, M. C. (2009). The
association between transfer of emergency department boarders to inpatient hallways and mortality: a 4-year experience. Annals of emergency medicine, 54(4), 487-491.

Wikipedia: The Free Encyclopedia. (2014). Emergency department. Wikimedia

Foundation, Inc. Retrieved from http://en.wikipedia.org/wiki/Emergency_department

Wiler, J. L., Griffey, R. T. and Olsen, T. (2011). Review of modeling approaches for
emergency department patient flow and crowding research. Academic Emergency Medicine, 18: 1371–1379. doi: 10.1111/j.1553-2712.2011.01135.x

Appendix A: Survey Questionnaire Tool

1. Participants and legal guardians have the right to obtain results of study upon request.

Consent statement: The individual signing this informed consent, participants or the individuals' legal guardian agree to participate in the research project.

Agree
Disagree

2. Do you feel patient flow in emergency departments are a problem?

Yes
No

3. How likely is it that the cause of emergency department overcrowding is from decreased patient flow through the department?

Very Likely
Moderately Likely
Slightly Likely
Not at all Likely

4. Has patient flow in emergency departments become a problem due to the lack of patients not having medical insurance related to the bad economy and high unemployment rates?

Completely True
Very True
Moderately True
Slightly True
Not at all True

5. Do you think most barriers slowing down patient flow in emergency departments lies only within the department?

Yes
No

6. Does admitted patients residing in the emergency department, waiting on inpatient beds, decrease patient flow through the department?

Extremely Influential
Moderately Influential
Slightly Influential
Not at all Influential

7. Can patient flow in emergency departments be affected by hospital census?

Yes
No

8. Is quality care and patient safety negatively affected by decreased patient flow through emergency departments?

Always
Often
Sometimes
Rarely
Never

9. Which barrier(s) is the most likely cause of negative affects on patient flow through emergency departments? (Select all that apply)

Admitted patients in ED
Waiting on lab results
Waiting on radiology results
Not enough inpatient beds
Not enough staff available
Other (please specify)

www.ingramcontent.com/pod-product-compliance
Lightning Source LLC
Chambersburg PA
CBHW030548220526
45463CB00007B/3026